SMOOTHIES FOR CANCER

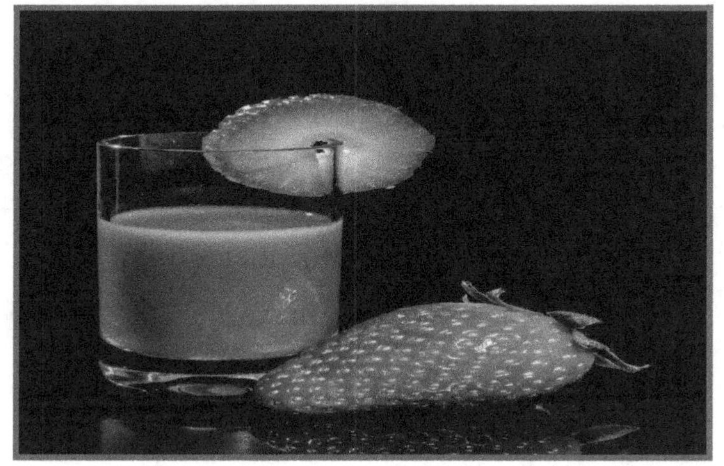

Nutrient-Packed Blends for Wellness

Karla Mayer

Table Of Contents

Introduction

In the battle against cancer, one of the most overlooked yet powerful allies is nutrition. The foods we consume play a critical role in our overall health, and this is especially true when it comes to combating cancer. Among the many nutritional strategies available, smoothies stand out as a versatile, delicious, and effective way to deliver vital nutrients to the body. This book, "Smoothies for Cancer," aims to empower individuals with knowledge and practical recipes that harness the healing power of smoothies.

Cancer is a complex and multifaceted disease, affecting millions of people worldwide. While medical treatments such as chemotherapy, radiation, and surgery are essential in fighting cancer, complementary approaches like nutrition can significantly enhance the body's ability to cope with these treatments and improve overall well-being. Smoothies, in particular, offer a unique advantage because they are easy to prepare, can be packed with a variety of nutrient-dense ingredients, and are generally easy on the digestive system.

The connection between diet and cancer prevention or recovery is supported by extensive research. Many fruits, vegetables, and other natural ingredients contain compounds known for their cancer-fighting properties. For instance, berries are rich in antioxidants, leafy greens are packed with vitamins and minerals, and nuts and seeds offer healthy fats and proteins. By blending these ingredients into smoothies, we can create potent nutritional blends that support the body's defenses and aid in recovery.

This book is organized into eight chapters, each focusing on different aspects of incorporating smoothies into a cancer-fighting diet. We begin by exploring the scientific foundation of how nutrition impacts cancer, providing a solid understanding of why what we eat matters. From there, we delve into the specific benefits of smoothies, highlighting their convenience and effectiveness in delivering concentrated doses of nutrients.

The chapters on essential ingredients and superfoods will introduce you to a variety of powerful foods that should be staples in your smoothie recipes. You'll learn about fruits and vegetables that are particularly effective in fighting cancer, as well as other superfoods like chia seeds, turmeric, and green tea, which can enhance the nutritional profile of your smoothies.

Creating the perfect smoothie requires a balance of macronutrients (carbohydrates, proteins, and fats) and micronutrients (vitamins and minerals). We will guide you through the process of building balanced smoothies that not only taste great but also provide comprehensive nutritional support. Additionally, we will discuss the importance of detoxification and how specific smoothie recipes can help cleanse the body of toxins, potentially reducing the burden on your immune system.

A strong immune system is crucial for anyone battling cancer. Our chapter on immunity-boosting smoothies focuses on ingredients that can help strengthen your body's natural defenses. Moreover, recognizing that different types of cancer may benefit from different nutritional strategies, we offer tailored smoothie recipes that address the unique needs of various cancer types.

For those undergoing cancer treatment or in recovery, nutrition plays a critical role in maintaining strength and promoting healing. We provide a selection of recipes designed to support you during these challenging times, helping to manage treatment side effects and accelerate recovery. Finally, we emphasize the importance of making smoothies a part of your daily routine, not just as a temporary measure but as a sustainable, healthy lifestyle choice.

"Smoothies for Cancer" is more than just a recipe book; it is a comprehensive guide to using nutrition as a powerful tool in the fight against cancer. Whether you are a patient, a caregiver, or someone looking to reduce your cancer risk, this book offers valuable insights and practical solutions to help you harness the healing power of smoothies. Join us on this journey to better health, one smoothie at a time.

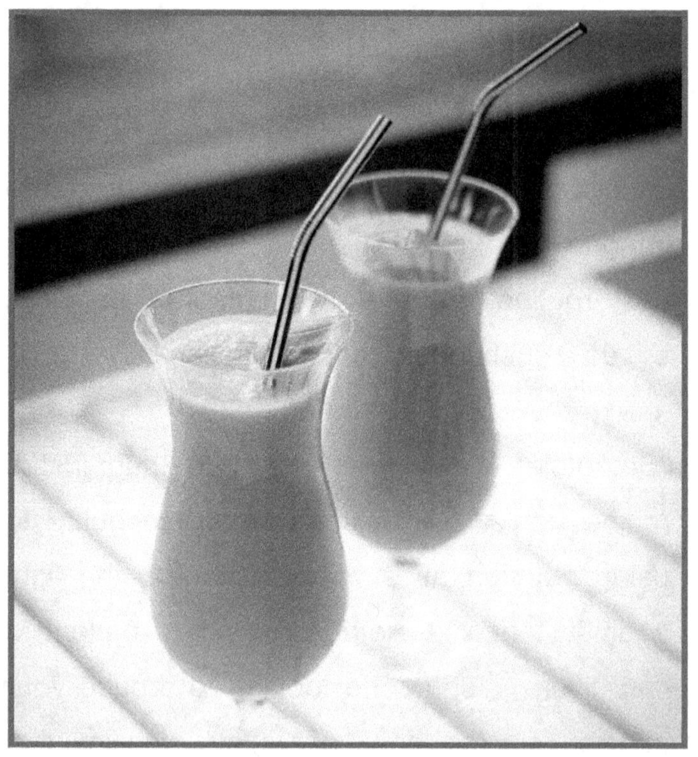

Chapter One

The Power of Nutrition in Cancer Prevention and Management

Nutrition plays a crucial role in both the prevention and management of cancer. What we eat can significantly impact our overall health, influence the risk of developing cancer, and aid in the body's ability to fight the disease. While no single food or diet can prevent cancer, a balanced, nutrient-rich diet can support the immune system, maintain a healthy weight, and provide the body with essential vitamins and minerals. One delicious and effective way to incorporate these beneficial nutrients into your diet is through smoothies.

Why Smoothies?

Smoothies are an excellent way to consume a variety of fruits, vegetables, and other nutrient-dense ingredients in a convenient and tasty format. They can be customized to include specific ingredients known for their cancer-fighting properties and are easy to digest, which is particularly beneficial for individuals undergoing cancer treatment who may have difficulties with solid foods.

Key Ingredients for Cancer-Fighting Smoothies

Leafy Greens: Spinach, kale, and other greens are high in vitamins, minerals, and antioxidants. They contain chlorophyll, which can help detoxify the body, and compounds like sulforaphane that have been shown to inhibit cancer cell growth.

Berries: Blueberries, strawberries, and raspberries are high in antioxidants such as vitamin C and anthocyanins. These antioxidants help protect cells from damage caused by free radicals, which can lead to cancer.

Cruciferous Vegetables: Broccoli, cauliflower, and Brussels sprouts are known for their high content of glucosinolates, compounds that may help reduce the risk of certain cancers.

Healthy Fats: Ingredients like avocado, flaxseeds, and chia seeds provide essential omega-3 fatty acids, which have anti-inflammatory properties and may help reduce cancer risk.

Turmeric and Ginger: Both spices have potent anti-inflammatory and antioxidant effects. Curcumin, the active compound in turmeric, has been studied for its potential to inhibit cancer cell growth and metastasis.

Green Tea: Adding a splash of brewed green tea to your smoothie can boost its cancer-fighting power. Green tea contains catechins, which are powerful antioxidants that may help prevent cancer cell growth.

Sample Smoothie Recipes

Berry Green Detox Smoothie

1 cup spinach

1 cup mixed berries (blueberries, strawberries, raspberries)

1 banana

1 tablespoon chia seeds

1 cup unsweetened almond milk

1 teaspoon honey (optional)

Blend all ingredients until smooth and enjoy

Tropical Turmeric Smoothie

1 cup frozen pineapple chunks

1 cup coconut water

1 small avocado

1 teaspoon turmeric

1 teaspoon ginger (fresh or powdered)

1 tablespoon flaxseeds

Blend all ingredients until smooth and enjoy!

The Role of Smoothies During Cancer Treatment

Cancer treatments such as chemotherapy and radiation can lead to various side effects, including nausea, loss of appetite, and difficulty swallowing. Smoothies can provide a palatable and nutritious option for patients who struggle with these symptoms. They offer a way to consume calories and essential nutrients without overwhelming the digestive system.

Personalized Nutrition
It's important to note that individual nutritional needs can vary greatly, especially for cancer patients. Consulting with a healthcare provider or a registered dietitian who specializes in oncology nutrition can help tailor smoothie

recipes and overall diet plans to meet specific needs and support treatment goals.

Incorporating nutrient-rich smoothies into your diet can be a delicious and effective way to support your health, whether you're looking to reduce your cancer risk or manage your nutrition during treatment. By understanding the connection between nutrition and cancer, you can make informed choices that contribute to your overall well-being.

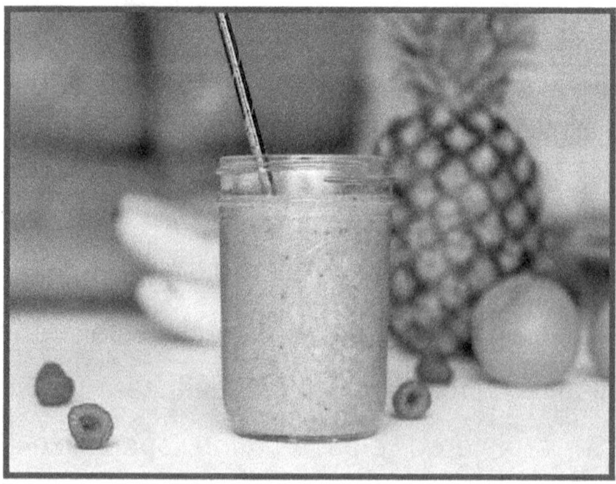

Chapter Two

The Science Behind Smoothies: A Nutritional Powerhouse

Nutrition is a cornerstone of health, playing a pivotal role in preventing and managing diseases, including cancer. While no single food can cure cancer, a diet rich in a variety of nutrients can support the body's natural defenses, reduce inflammation, and improve overall well-being. This is where smoothies come in—they are an easy, delicious way to pack a nutritional punch, especially beneficial for those battling cancer.

Why Smoothies Are Ideal

Smoothies are a fantastic way to incorporate a wide array of nutrients into a single, easy-to-consume meal or snack. They are particularly beneficial for cancer patients who might have trouble eating solid foods due to treatment side effects like nausea, mouth sores, or difficulty swallowing. By blending fruits, vegetables, and other healthful ingredients, smoothies can provide essential vitamins, minerals, antioxidants, and fiber in a form that's gentle on the digestive system.

Key Nutrients in Cancer-Fighting Smoothies

1. Antioxidants

Antioxidants are compounds that protect cells from damage caused by free radicals, which are unstable molecules that can cause oxidative stress and lead to cancer. Smoothies packed with fruits and vegetables are rich in antioxidants like vitamin C, vitamin E, and beta-carotene.

Berries: Blueberries, strawberries, and raspberries are antioxidant powerhouses. They contain vitamins C and E and compounds like anthocyanins, which have been shown to reduce oxidative stress and inflammation.

Leafy Greens: Spinach, kale, and Swiss chard are high in antioxidants like vitamin C, vitamin E, and beta-carotene.

2. Phytochemicals

Phytochemicals are naturally occurring compounds in plants that have been shown to have cancer-fighting properties. They include flavonoids, polyphenols, and glucosinolates.

Cruciferous Vegetables: Broccoli, cauliflower, and Brussels sprouts contain glucosinolates, which can help detoxify carcinogens and inhibit the growth of cancer cells.

Green Tea: Rich in catechins, green tea can be added to smoothies to provide a potent dose of these cancer-fighting phytochemicals.

3. Fiber

Dietary fiber is essential for maintaining a healthy digestive system and has been linked to a reduced risk of colorectal cancer. It aids in the regulation of the body's sugar consumption, hence controlling appetite and blood sugar levels.

Oats and Flaxseeds: These can be added to smoothies to boost fiber content. Flaxseeds also include omega-3 fatty acids, which have an anti-inflammatory effect.

Fruits and Vegetables: Most fruits and vegetables are excellent sources of dietary fiber.

4. Healthy Fats

Healthy fats are essential for good health and can assist to minimize inflammation. Omega-3 fatty acids, in particular, have been studied for their potential role in cancer prevention.

Avocado: This adds creaminess to smoothies and provides healthy monounsaturated fats.

Chia Seeds: These tiny seeds include omega-3 fatty acids, fiber, and protein.

5. Protein

Adequate protein intake is essential for maintaining muscle mass and supporting the immune system, especially during cancer treatment.

Greek Yogurt: This adds creaminess and a protein boost to smoothies.

Nut Butters: Almond or peanut butter can add protein and healthy fats.

Sample Smoothie Recipes

Berry Antioxidant Blast

1 cup mixed berries (blueberries, strawberries, raspberries)

1 cup spinach

1 banana

1 tablespoon chia seeds

1 cup unsweetened almond milk

1 teaspoon honey (optional)

Blend all ingredients until smooth.

Green Power Smoothie

1 cup kale

1 small avocado

1 green apple

1 cup green tea (cooled)

1 tablespoon flaxseeds

1 teaspoon fresh ginger

Blend all ingredients until smooth.

Smoothies During Cancer Treatment

Cancer treatments such as chemotherapy and radiation can lead to side effects that make eating challenging. Smoothies are a practical solution, providing a way to consume essential nutrients without the discomfort of chewing or digesting solid food. They can be tailored to meet individual dietary needs and preferences, ensuring that patients receive adequate nutrition to support their treatment and recovery.

Smoothies offer a powerful and versatile way to boost nutrition, particularly for those dealing with cancer. By understanding the science behind the ingredients and their potential benefits, you can create delicious, nutrient-dense smoothies that support overall health and complement cancer treatment. Remember, the key to the best outcomes is a balanced diet, personalized nutrition, and professional guidance tailored to individual needs and preferences.

Chapter Three

Essential Ingredients: Fruits and Vegetables with Cancer-Fighting Properties

Nutrition plays a vital role in our health, and when it comes to preventing and managing cancer, certain fruits and vegetables stand out due to their powerful cancer-fighting properties. These foods are packed with essential nutrients, antioxidants, and phytochemicals that can help reduce the risk of cancer and support the body's natural defenses. Let's dive into some of the most potent cancer-fighting fruits and vegetables and understand how they contribute to a healthier you.

Fruits with Cancer-Fighting Properties

1. Berries

Berries such as blueberries, strawberries, raspberries, and blackberries are among the top fruits for their cancer-fighting potential. They are rich in vitamins, minerals, and antioxidants like vitamin C, ellagic acid, and anthocyanins, which help protect cells from damage.

Blueberries: High in antioxidants, blueberries can neutralize free radicals, reducing oxidative stress and inflammation, both of which are linked to cancer development.

Strawberries: These berries contain ellagic acid, a compound that has been shown to prevent the growth of cancer cells in the laboratory.

Raspberries: Particularly rich in fiber, vitamins, and antioxidants, raspberries have compounds that may inhibit cancer cell proliferation.

2. Citrus Fruits

Citrus fruits such as oranges, lemons, limes, and grapefruits are excellent sources of vitamin C and flavonoids, both of which have been linked to cancer prevention.

Oranges: Packed with vitamin C and flavonoids, oranges help boost the immune system and protect cells from damage.

Lemons and Limes: High in limonoids and flavonoids, these fruits can help detoxify the body and inhibit cancer cell growth.

Grapefruits: Rich in lycopene (especially pink grapefruits), they offer antioxidant properties that help protect against cancer.

3. Apples

"An apple a day keeps the doctor away" holds some truth, especially when it comes to cancer prevention. Apples are high in fiber, vitamin C, and various phytochemicals.

Quercetin: A flavonoid found in apples that has been shown to inhibit cancer cell growth.

Pectin: A type of fiber in apples that helps detoxify the body and may reduce the risk of colon cancer.

4. Pomegranates
Pomegranates are loaded with polyphenols and anthocyanins, powerful antioxidants that have anti-inflammatory and anti-cancer properties.

Ellagic Acid: This compound found in pomegranates helps inhibit the growth of cancer cells and deactivates cancer-causing compounds.

Vegetables with Cancer-Fighting Properties

1. Cruciferous Vegetables

Cruciferous vegetables like broccoli, cauliflower, Brussels sprouts, and kale are well-known for their cancer-fighting properties due to their high content of glucosinolates.

Broccoli: Contains sulforaphane, a compound that has been shown to kill cancer stem cells and slow tumor growth.

Cauliflower: Rich in glucosinolates and isothiocyanates, which can detoxify carcinogens and reduce cancer risk.

Brussels Sprouts: These mini cabbages contain high levels of glucosinolates and can enhance the body's detoxification processes.

Kale: Known as a superfood, kale is loaded with vitamins, minerals, and antioxidants, including sulforaphane and indole-3-carbinol, which have anti-cancer effects.

2. Leafy Greens

Leafy greens such as spinach, Swiss chard, and collard greens are nutritional powerhouses rich in vitamins, minerals, and antioxidants.

Spinach: High in lutein, zeaxanthin, and beta-carotene, which protect cells from damage and reduce cancer risk.

Swiss Chard: Contains syringic acid, which has been shown to prevent the growth of cancer cells.

Collard Greens: Rich in antioxidants and fiber, helping to cleanse the digestive tract and prevent cancer.

3. Tomatoes

Tomatoes are a great source of lycopene, an antioxidant linked to a reduced risk of prostate, lung, and stomach cancers.

Lycopene: This powerful antioxidant gives tomatoes their red color and has been shown to protect cells from damage and slow cancer cell growth.

4. Garlic and Onions

Garlic and onions belong to the allium family and are known for their immune-boosting and cancer-fighting properties.

Garlic: Contains allicin, which has been shown to reduce the risk of stomach and colorectal cancers.

Onions: Rich in sulfur compounds and flavonoids, onions can help detoxify carcinogens and prevent cancer cell growth.

How to Include These Foods into Your Diet

Incorporating these cancer-fighting fruits and vegetables into your diet doesn't have to be difficult. Here are some tips:

Smoothies: Blend a mix of berries, spinach, kale, and a splash of citrus juice for a nutrient-packed smoothie.

Salads: Create colorful salads with leafy greens, tomatoes, cruciferous vegetables, and a lemon-based dressing.

Snacks: Enjoy apple slices with a nut butter dip or a handful of mixed berries as a snack.

Cooking: Add garlic and onions to your favorite dishes, stir-fries, or soups for an added health boost.

Juicing: Make fresh juices combining pomegranates, citrus fruits, and leafy greens for a refreshing and healthy drink.

Including a variety of fruits and vegetables with cancer-fighting properties into your diet is a powerful way to support your health and reduce cancer risk. By understanding the benefits of these foods and finding creative ways to include them in your meals, you can make a significant impact on your overall well-being. Remember, the key is diversity and consistency in your diet, ensuring you get a broad spectrum of nutrients to help your body stay strong and healthy.

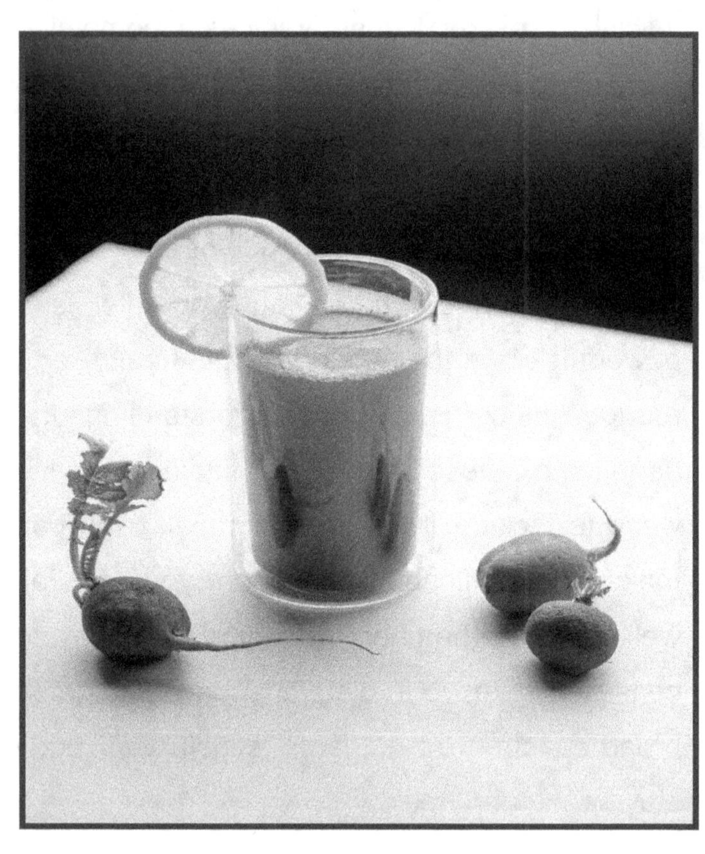

Chapter Four

Superfoods to Include in Your Smoothies

Smoothies are a convenient and delicious way to pack a lot of nutrition into one easy-to-consume meal. When it comes to cancer prevention and management, choosing the right ingredients for your smoothies can make a significant difference. Superfoods, known for their high nutrient content and potential health benefits, are particularly powerful additions to your smoothie recipes. Here's an extensive look at some superfoods you should consider including in your smoothies to support your health and fight cancer.

Leafy Greens

1. Spinach

Spinach is a nutrient-dense leafy green packed with vitamins, minerals, and antioxidants. It contains high levels of vitamins A, C, and K, as well as folate, iron, and calcium.

Benefits: Spinach is rich in lutein and zeaxanthin, which are antioxidants that protect cells from damage and reduce inflammation. It also contains chlorophyll, which helps the body detoxify from carcinogens.

2. Kale

Kale is often touted as a superfood because of its impressive nutrient profile. It contains high levels of vitamins A, C, and K, along with minerals like calcium and potassium.

Benefits: Kale is particularly high in sulforaphane, a compound that has been shown to inhibit cancer cell growth. It also contains indole-3-carbinol, which helps in DNA repair and may block the growth of cancer cells.

Berries

3. Blueberries

Blueberries are among the most antioxidant-rich fruits. They are high in vitamins C and K and contain fiber and manganese.

Benefits: The high levels of anthocyanins in blueberries help fight oxidative stress and inflammation, both of which are linked to cancer development. They also have been shown to inhibit the growth of cancer cells in various studies.

4. Strawberries

Strawberries are loaded with vitamins, fiber, and particularly high levels of antioxidants like vitamin C and ellagic acid.

Benefits: Ellagic acid in strawberries has been found to prevent skin, bladder, lung, and esophageal cancers. Strawberries also have anti-inflammatory properties that can reduce the risk of chronic diseases, including cancer.

Seeds and Nuts

5. Flaxseeds

Flaxseeds are tiny powerhouses of nutrition, rich in omega-3 fatty acids, fiber, and lignans, which are phytoestrogens with antioxidant properties.

Benefits: The lignans in flaxseeds have been shown to reduce the growth of hormone-related cancers such as breast cancer. They also help in reducing inflammation and regulating hormones.

6. Chia Seeds

Chia seeds are packed with omega-3 fatty acids, fiber, protein, and various essential minerals like calcium, magnesium, and phosphorus.

Benefits: The high fiber content aids in digestion and helps to remove toxins from the body, potentially lowering the risk of colorectal cancer. Omega-3s in chia seeds also have anti-inflammatory properties.

Other Superfoods

7. Turmeric

Turmeric is a vibrant yellow spice that contains curcumin, a compound known for its potent anti-inflammatory and antioxidant effects.

Benefits: Curcumin has been extensively studied for its ability to reduce the growth of cancer cells and inhibit the spread of tumors. It also enhances the body's antioxidant capacity.

8. Green Tea

Green tea is rich in catechins, particularly epigallocatechin gallate (EGCG), which is a powerful antioxidant.

Benefits: The antioxidants in green tea can help protect cells from DNA damage and inhibit the growth of cancer cells. Green tea also boosts metabolism and aids in detoxification.

9. Ginger

Ginger is a root known for its medicinal properties and is packed with antioxidants and anti-inflammatory compounds.

Benefits: Ginger has been shown to reduce inflammation and may slow the growth of cancer cells. It also helps alleviate nausea, a common side effect of cancer treatments.

10. Pomegranate

Pomegranates are rich in polyphenols, particularly punicalagins and anthocyanins, which have strong antioxidant properties.

Benefits: Pomegranate compounds have been shown to inhibit the growth of cancer cells and reduce inflammation. They also support heart health and overall well-being.

Sample Smoothie Recipes

Green Detox Smoothie

1 cup spinach

1 cup kale

1 banana

1 tablespoon flaxseeds

1 cup unsweetened almond milk

1 teaspoon turmeric

Blend all ingredients until smooth.

Berry Antioxidant Smoothie

1 cup mixed berries (blueberries, strawberries, raspberries)

1 cup green tea (cooled)

1 tablespoon chia seeds

1 teaspoon fresh ginger

1 tablespoon pomegranate seeds

Blend all ingredients until smooth.

Including these superfoods in your smoothies can provide a wide range of nutrients that support overall health and help fight cancer. By incorporating a variety of leafy greens, berries, seeds, nuts, and other powerful ingredients like turmeric, green tea, and ginger, you can create delicious and nutritious smoothies that contribute to your well-being. Remember, while superfoods are a fantastic addition to a healthy diet, they should be part of a balanced and varied diet to ensure you get all the necessary nutrients your body needs.

Chapter Five

Building a Balanced Smoothie: Macronutrients and Micronutrients

Smoothies are not just a tasty treat; they can be a nutritional powerhouse, especially for those looking to prevent or manage cancer. To maximize their health benefits, it's essential to create a balanced smoothie that includes both macronutrients and micronutrients. This balance ensures that you get the energy you need while also providing your body with the vitamins and minerals crucial for health and healing. Let's explore how to build a balanced smoothie that is both delicious and nutritionally complete.

The Basics of Macronutrients

Macronutrients are the nutrients that our bodies need in larger amounts: carbohydrates, proteins, and fats. Each plays a vital role in maintaining health and supporting bodily functions.

1. Carbohydrates

Carbohydrates are the body's primary energy source. They are broken down into glucose, which fuels our cells. Including healthy carbohydrates in your smoothie can help maintain energy levels, especially important during cancer treatment.

Fruits: Bananas, berries, apples, and mangoes are excellent sources of natural sugars and fiber.

Vegetables: Spinach, kale, and carrots provide complex carbohydrates along with essential vitamins and minerals.

Grains: Oats and quinoa can add a hearty dose of fiber and sustained energy.

2. Proteins

Proteins are essential for building and repairing tissues, making them particularly important for cancer patients who may be dealing with muscle loss or other tissue damage from treatments.

Greek Yogurt: High in protein and probiotics, it adds creaminess to smoothies.

Protein Powders: Whey, pea, or hemp protein powders can boost the protein content.

Nut Butters: Almond butter, peanut butter, or sunflower seed butter add protein and healthy fats.

3. Fats

Healthy fats are crucial for absorbing fat-soluble vitamins (A, D, E, K) and providing long-lasting energy. They also have anti-inflammatory properties, which can be beneficial for cancer patients.

Avocado provides a creamy mouthfeel and is high in monounsaturated fats.

Seeds: Chia seeds, flaxseeds, and hemp seeds are packed with omega-3 fatty acids.

Nuts: Almonds, walnuts, and cashews provide healthy fats and a bit of protein.

The Importance of Micronutrients

Micronutrients, including vitamins and minerals, are needed in smaller amounts but are crucial for nearly every bodily function. They support the immune system, help in cell repair, and provide antioxidant protection.

1. Vitamins

Vitamins are chemical substances that are essential to health. They support everything from the immune system to vision and skin health.

Vitamin C: Found in citrus fruits, strawberries, and bell peppers, it's essential for immune function and skin health.

Vitamin A: Present in carrots, sweet potatoes, and leafy greens, it's important for vision and immune health.

B Vitamins: Bananas, avocados, and leafy greens provide these vitamins that help convert food into energy.

2. Minerals

Minerals like calcium, potassium, and magnesium are crucial for bone health, muscle function, and maintaining fluid balance.

Calcium: Found in dairy products, fortified plant milks, and leafy greens.

Bananas, oranges, and spinach are excellent sources, helping to regulate fluid balance and muscle contractions.

Magnesium: Present in nuts, seeds, and leafy greens, it supports muscle and nerve function.

Building Your Balanced Smoothie

Creating a balanced smoothie involves combining these macronutrients and micronutrients in a way that is both nutritious and tasty. Here's a step-by-step guide to building a smoothie that covers all your nutritional bases.

Step 1: Choose Your Base

The base of your smoothie adds liquid and can also contribute to the nutrient profile.

Water: Hydrating and calorie-free.

Plant-Based Milks: Almond milk, soy milk, and oat milk add creaminess and nutrients.

Green Tea: Adds antioxidants and a subtle flavor.

Step 2: Add Fruits and Vegetables

These provide essential vitamins, minerals, fiber, and natural sweetness.

Fruits: Aim for a mix of berries, bananas, and tropical fruits for a variety of nutrients.
Vegetables: Leafy greens like spinach and kale blend well and are nutrient-dense.

Step 3: Include Protein Sources
Protein helps keep you full and supports muscle and tissue repair.

Greek Yogurt: Adds creaminess and protein.
Protein Powder: Choose a high-quality protein powder that suits your dietary needs.
Nut Butters: A spoonful of almond or peanut butter for protein and healthy fats.

Step 4: Add Healthy Fats
Healthy fats are essential for nutrient absorption and overall health.

Avocado: Adds a smooth texture and healthy fats.

Seeds: Chia seeds, flaxseeds, or hemp seeds for omega-3 fatty acids.

Nuts: A handful of nuts for a protein and fat boost.

Step 5: Boost with Superfoods
Superfoods add an extra layer of nutrients and health benefits.

Turmeric: Anti-inflammatory properties.

Ginger: Aids digestion and has anti-inflammatory benefits.

Spirulina: A source of protein, vitamins, and minerals.

Sample Balanced Smoothie Recipe

Power Green Smoothie

Base: 1 cup unsweetened almond milk

Fruits: 1 banana, ½ cup frozen blueberries

Vegetables: 1 cup spinach, ½ cup kale

Protein: 1 scoop whey or pea protein powder

Healthy Fats: 1 tablespoon chia seeds, ¼ avocado

Superfoods: 1 teaspoon turmeric, 1 teaspoon spirulina

Optional Sweetener: 1 teaspoon honey or a date for natural sweetness

Instructions:

Add the almond milk to the blender.

Add the banana, blueberries, spinach, and kale.

Include the protein powder, chia seeds, and avocado.

Add turmeric and spirulina.

Blend until smooth. If needed, add more almond milk to achieve the desired consistency.

Taste and adjust sweetness with honey or a date if desired.
Enjoy immediately for the best flavor and nutritional benefit.

Building a balanced smoothie that includes a variety of macronutrients and micronutrients can provide comprehensive nutritional support, especially important for those dealing with cancer. By thoughtfully selecting your ingredients, you can create delicious smoothies that not only taste great but also help nourish your body, support your immune system, and promote overall health. Remember, the key to a great smoothie is balance, variety, and using fresh, high-quality ingredients.

Chapter Six

Smoothies for Different Stages

Cancer journeys are highly individual, with nutritional needs varying greatly depending on the stage of the disease and the type of treatment. Smoothies can be tailored to support these varying needs, providing essential nutrients in an easy-to-consume form. Here's a brief guide on creating smoothies for different stages of cancer.

Pre-Treatment Smoothies

Let's explore in detail the subject of pre-treatment smoothies for cancer patients. These specially designed smoothies can play a crucial role in preparing the body for the rigors of cancer treatment. Not only do they provide essential nutrients, but they also help manage symptoms and side effects, boost the immune system, and improve overall well-being.

Understanding Pre-Treatment Smoothies

When someone is about to undergo cancer treatment, such as chemotherapy, radiation, or surgery, their body needs to be in the best possible condition. Treatments can be tough, often leading to fatigue, nausea, and a weakened immune system. Pre-treatment smoothies are tailored to help mitigate these effects by:

Boosting Nutrient Intake: They are packed with vitamins, minerals, antioxidants, and other nutrients that are often needed in higher amounts during cancer treatment.

Supporting Immune Function: Ingredients like berries, leafy greens, and nuts are rich in immune-boosting properties.

Easing Digestion: Smoothies are easier to digest than solid foods, making them ideal for patients who might have difficulty eating due to stress or other pre-treatment factors.

Hydration: Many smoothie recipes include hydrating fruits and vegetables, which are essential since cancer treatments can lead to dehydration.

Key Ingredients in Pre-Treatment Smoothies

Here are some powerhouse ingredients commonly found in pre-treatment smoothies, along with their benefits:

Leafy Greens (Spinach, Kale): These are loaded with vitamins A, C, and K, folate, and fiber. They help to cleanse the body and boost the immune system

Berries (Blueberries, Strawberries, Raspberries): High in antioxidants, these fruits help protect cells from damage and inflammation.

Citrus Fruits (Oranges, Lemons): Rich in vitamin C, citrus fruits boost the immune system and enhance iron absorption.

Bananas: They provide a quick source of energy and are gentle on the stomach.

Nuts and Seeds (Almonds, Chia Seeds, Flaxseeds): Excellent sources of healthy fats, protein, and fiber, they support overall health and help maintain weight.

Ginger and Turmeric: Both have powerful anti-inflammatory and antioxidant properties, helping to reduce nausea and support immune health.

Yogurt or Kefir: These provide probiotics for gut health, which is important for nutrient absorption and immune function.

Sample Pre-Treatment Smoothie Recipes

1. Green Immunity Smoothie

Ingredients:

1 cup spinach

1/2 cup kale

1 green apple, cored and chopped

1/2 banana

1 tablespoon chia seeds

1 cup unsweetened almond milk

Juice of 1/2 lemon

Instructions:

Add all ingredients to a blender.

Blend until smooth.

Enjoy immediately.

2. Berry Antioxidant Blast

Ingredients:

1/2 cup blueberries

1/2 cup strawberries

1/2 cup raspberries

1/2 banana

1/2 cup plain Greek yogurt

1 tablespoon honey (optional)

1 cup water or coconut water

Instructions:

Combine all ingredients in a blender.

Blend until creamy and smooth.

Serve chilled.

3. Tropical Ginger Turmeric Smoothie

Ingredients:

1 cup pineapple chunks

1/2 mango, peeled and chopped

1 small carrot, peeled and chopped

1/2 teaspoon fresh ginger, grated

1/4 teaspoon turmeric powder

1 cup coconut water

Ice cubes (optional)

Instructions:

Place all ingredients in a blender.

Blend until smooth and frothy.

Drink immediately.

Tips for Making the Perfect Pre-Treatment Smoothie

Balance is Key: Aim for a good mix of fruits, vegetables, proteins, and healthy fats to ensure a balanced nutrient profile.

Customize to Taste: Feel free to adjust recipes according to your taste preferences and dietary restrictions.

Fresh and Organic: Whenever possible, use fresh, organic ingredients to minimize exposure to pesticides and maximize nutrient intake.

Listen to Your Body: Everyone's body reacts differently, so listen to what your body needs and tolerates well.

Consult Your Healthcare Team: Before making significant changes to your diet, it's important to discuss with your healthcare providers, especially when dealing with cancer.

The Emotional and Psychological Benefits

Preparing and consuming these smoothies can also have emotional and psychological benefits. The process of making a nutritious smoothie can be empowering, giving patients a sense of control over their health. Enjoying a delicious, colorful smoothie can also be a small but significant pleasure in the day, providing comfort and a sense of normalcy.

Pre-treatment smoothies for cancer patients are much more than just a blend of fruits and vegetables. They represent a holistic approach to health, offering vital nutrients, supporting the immune system, and providing both physical and emotional nourishment. By incorporating these smoothies into their routine, cancer patients can give their bodies a much-needed boost as they prepare for the challenging journey ahead.

During - Treatment Smoothies

These smoothies are designed specifically to meet the various dietary and symptom requirements that come up after cancer treatment. Chemotherapy, radiation, and surgery, among other therapies, can be extremely taxing on the body and cause a number of side effects that might affect general health and nutrition.

Importance of During-Treatment Smoothies

During cancer treatment, patients often face side effects such as nausea, loss of appetite, mouth sores, fatigue, and digestive issues. During-treatment smoothies can help manage these symptoms by:

Providing Easily Digestible Nutrition: Smoothies are easier to consume and digest than solid foods, which is crucial when dealing with nausea or digestive problems.

Offering High Nutrient Density: They can be packed with vitamins, minerals, antioxidants, and other essential nutrients to support the body's needs.

Maintaining Hydration: Many smoothies have high water content from fruits and vegetables, which is essential for staying hydrated, especially when treatments can lead to dehydration.

Enhancing Energy Levels: They provide a quick source of energy through natural sugars and carbohydrates, helping to combat fatigue.

Key Ingredients in During-Treatment Smoothies

Let's explore some of the best ingredients to include in during-treatment smoothies and their benefits:

Bananas: Gentle on the stomach, bananas provide a good source of energy and potassium, which can help with muscle cramps and overall energy levels.

Berries (Blueberries, Strawberries, Raspberries): Rich in antioxidants, these can help protect the body's cells from damage and boost the immune system.

Ginger: Known for its anti-nausea properties, ginger can help reduce the feeling of sickness often caused by treatments.

Yogurt or Kefir: These are excellent sources of probiotics, which support gut health and can help with digestive issues.

Oats: Adding oats provides soluble fiber, which can help with digestive health and sustain energy levels.

Nut Butters (Almond, Peanut, Cashew): High in healthy fats and protein, nut butters can help maintain weight and provide essential nutrients.

Leafy Greens (Spinach, Kale): These are packed with vitamins A, C, K, and folate, which support overall health and immune function.

Avocado: Offers healthy fats and a creamy texture, making smoothies more filling and providing essential nutrients.

Sample During-Treatment Smoothie Recipes

1. Creamy Banana Ginger Smoothie

Ingredients:

1 banana

1/2 cup plain Greek yogurt

1/2 teaspoon fresh ginger, grated

1 tablespoon honey

1 cup almond milk

Ice cubes (optional)

Instructions:

Combine all ingredients in a blender.

Blend until smooth and creamy.

Serve immediately.

2. Berry Gut-Health Smoothie

Ingredients:

1/2 cup blueberries

1/2 cup strawberries

1/2 cup raspberries

1/2 cup plain kefir or yogurt

1 tablespoon chia seeds

1 cup coconut water

Instructions:

Place all ingredients in a blender.

Blend until smooth.

Enjoy chilled.

3. Nutty Green Energy Smoothie

Ingredients:

1 cup spinach

1/2 avocado

1 banana

1 tablespoon almond butter

1 cup oat milk

1 tablespoon honey or maple syrup (optional)

Instructions:

Add all ingredients to a blender.

Blend until smooth and well combined.

Drink immediately.

Tips for Making the Perfect During-Treatment Smoothie

Focus on Tolerance: Be mindful of what ingredients are well-tolerated. Some patients may have aversions or sensitivities during treatment.

Keep it Mild: Strong flavors or acidic ingredients can be harsh on a sensitive stomach or mouth sores.

Blend Thoroughly: Ensure smoothies are well-blended to avoid any chunks that might be difficult to swallow.

Adjust Consistency: Depending on preference and tolerance, adjust the thickness of the smoothie by adding more or less liquid.

Emotional and Psychological Benefits

Smoothies can offer more than just physical nourishment. The act of making and drinking a smoothie can provide a sense of routine and normalcy during a tumultuous time. The vibrant colors and refreshing tastes can also be a small, comforting pleasure, contributing positively to a patient's emotional well-being.

During-treatment smoothies for cancer patients are a valuable tool in managing the nutritional and symptomatic challenges posed by cancer treatments. These nutrient-dense, easily digestible beverages not only help maintain health and energy but also offer a comforting and enjoyable way to support the body during this critical time. By incorporating thoughtfully chosen ingredients and tailoring recipes to individual needs and preferences, these smoothies can make a significant positive impact on a patient's treatment journey.

Post-Treatment Smoothies

Just as the name implies, these smoothies are specifically designed to aid recovery after the completion of cancer treatment, helping to rebuild strength, restore energy, and support the body's return to normalcy. Post-treatment smoothies can play a vital role in healing and long-term health maintenance.

The Importance of Post-Treatment Smoothies

After completing cancer treatment, the body often needs to recover from the intense stress it has endured. Treatments like chemotherapy and radiation can leave lasting effects such as fatigue, weakened immunity, digestive issues, and nutritional deficiencies. Post-treatment smoothies can address these needs by:

Restoring Nutrient Levels: After treatment, the body may be depleted of essential vitamins and minerals. Smoothies can be packed with nutrient-dense ingredients to replenish these stores.

Supporting Immune Function: Ingredients high in antioxidants and other immune-boosting properties can help strengthen the immune system.

Promoting Healing and Repair: Smoothies can include ingredients that support tissue repair and overall healing.

Boosting Energy Levels: Natural sugars, proteins, and healthy fats in smoothies provide sustained energy, helping to combat post-treatment fatigue.

Improving Digestion: Smoothies are gentle on the digestive system and can include ingredients that promote gut health, which is often compromised during treatment.

Key Ingredients in Post-Treatment Smoothies

Here are some powerhouse ingredients to consider for post-treatment smoothies and their benefits:

Leafy Greens (Spinach, Kale): Rich in vitamins A, C, and K, as well as folate and iron, these greens support immune function and cellular repair.

Berries (Blueberries, Strawberries, Raspberries): High in antioxidants, which help fight free radicals and reduce inflammation.

Citrus Fruits (Oranges, Lemons, Limes): Packed with vitamin C, which boosts the immune system and aids in collagen production for tissue repair.

Avocado: Provides healthy fats, fiber, and vitamins E and B, all of which are essential for overall health and energy.

Greek Yogurt or Kefir: These offer probiotics for gut health, as well as protein and calcium for muscle and bone strength.

Nut Butters (Almond, Peanut, Cashew): High in healthy fats and protein, nut butters help in maintaining weight and muscle mass.

Flaxseeds and Chia Seeds: Excellent sources of omega-3 fatty acids, fiber, and antioxidants, supporting heart health and reducing inflammation.

Turmeric and Ginger: Both have strong anti-inflammatory and antioxidant properties, aiding in reducing post-treatment inflammation and boosting immunity.

Oats: Provide soluble fiber, which supports digestion and helps maintain energy levels.

Sample Post-Treatment Smoothie Recipes
1. Revitalizing Green Smoothie
Ingredients:

1 cup spinach

1/2 avocado

1 banana

1/2 cup Greek yogurt

1 tablespoon chia seeds

1 cup unsweetened almond milk

Juice of 1/2 lemon

Instructions:

Combine all ingredients in a blender.

Blend until smooth.

Enjoy immediately.

2. Berry Immune Booster

Ingredients:

1/2 cup blueberries

1/2 cup strawberries

1/2 cup raspberries

1/2 cup plain kefir

1 tablespoon flaxseeds

1 cup orange juice

Instructions:

Place all ingredients in a blender.

Blend until smooth.

Serve chilled.

3. Turmeric Ginger Recovery Smoothie

Ingredients:

1 cup mango chunks

1/2 cup pineapple chunks

1 small carrot, peeled and chopped

1/2 teaspoon fresh ginger, grated

1/4 teaspoon turmeric powder

1 cup coconut water

Instructions:

Add all ingredients to a blender.

Blend until smooth.

Drink immediately.

Tips for Making the Perfect Post-Treatment Smoothie

Prioritize Fresh, Organic Ingredients: This ensures maximum nutrient intake and reduces exposure to pesticides.

Focus on Balance: Aim for a good mix of fruits, vegetables, proteins, and healthy fats to provide a well-rounded nutrient profile.

Listen to Your Body: Adjust recipes based on what feels good and what your body tolerates well.

Keep it Simple: Sometimes, simpler smoothies are easier to digest and just as nutritious.

Stay Hydrated: Consider adding hydrating ingredients like coconut water or water-rich fruits and vegetables.

Emotional and Psychological Benefits

Post-treatment smoothies can also offer emotional and psychological benefits. Preparing and enjoying a nutritious smoothie can be a positive, comforting routine. The act of making a smoothie can be therapeutic, providing a sense of control and accomplishment. Additionally, the vibrant colors and fresh flavors can lift spirits and provide a small but meaningful pleasure during the recovery process.

Post-treatment smoothies for cancer patients are much more than just a tasty beverage. They are a powerful tool in the journey of recovery, providing essential nutrients, supporting immune function, and promoting overall healing. By thoughtfully selecting ingredients and tailoring recipes to individual needs and preferences, these smoothies can significantly enhance a patient's post-treatment experience, helping them regain strength, energy, and well-being.

Smoothies for Remission

Let's explore the topic of smoothies for remission in cancer care. These smoothies are specially designed to support ongoing health and prevent recurrence after the initial battle with cancer is won. Staying in remission requires maintaining a balanced diet, strengthening the immune system, and promoting overall wellness, and smoothies can be a delightful and effective part of that journey.

Understanding the Role of Smoothies in Remission

When a cancer patient reaches remission, it means that the signs and symptoms of cancer are reduced or undetectable. This is a significant milestone, but maintaining remission involves ongoing vigilance about one's health. Incorporating smoothies into a daily routine can provide several benefits:

Nutrient Density: Smoothies can be loaded with vitamins, minerals, antioxidants, and phytonutrients that help keep the body strong and resilient.

Immune Support: Ingredients rich in antioxidants and anti-inflammatory compounds can help bolster the immune system.

Detoxification: Smoothies can include ingredients that support liver function and help detoxify the body.

Energy and Vitality: They can provide a natural energy boost, helping to maintain a vibrant and active lifestyle.

Convenience and Enjoyment: Smoothies are quick to prepare, customizable, and delicious, making it easier to stick to a healthy diet.

Key Ingredients for Remission Smoothies

Let's highlight some powerful ingredients that are particularly beneficial for individuals in remission:

Leafy Greens (Spinach, Kale, Swiss Chard): These are packed with vitamins A, C, and K, iron, and fiber. They support detoxification and provide essential nutrients for overall health.

Berries (Blueberries, Strawberries, Acai): High in antioxidants, these help protect cells from damage and reduce inflammation.

Cruciferous Vegetables (Broccoli, Cauliflower): These contain compounds like sulforaphane that have been shown to have anti-cancer properties.

Citrus Fruits (Oranges, Grapefruits): Rich in vitamin C, these fruits boost the immune system and aid in collagen production.

Turmeric and Ginger: Both have strong anti-inflammatory and antioxidant effects, helping to maintain a healthy immune response.
Flaxseeds and Chia Seeds: Excellent sources of omega-3 fatty acids and fiber, which support heart health and digestion.

Nuts and Seeds (Almonds, Walnuts, Pumpkin Seeds): These provide healthy fats, protein, and essential vitamins and minerals.

Green Tea or Matcha: These are rich in catechins, which have powerful antioxidant effects.

Probiotics (Yogurt, Kefir): These support gut health, which is crucial for overall immunity and nutrient absorption.

Sample Remission Smoothie Recipes

1. Green Detox Smoothie

Ingredients:
1 cup spinach
1/2 cucumber, chopped

1 green apple, cored and chopped

1/2 avocado

1 tablespoon chia seeds

1 cup green tea (cooled)

Juice of 1/2 lemon

Instructions:

Combine all ingredients in a blender.

Blend until smooth.

Serve immediately.

2. Berry Antioxidant Smoothie

Ingredients:

1/2 cup blueberries

1/2 cup strawberries

1/2 cup acai berries (or acai puree)

1 tablespoon flaxseeds

1/2 cup plain Greek yogurt

1 cup almond milk

Instructions:

Place all ingredients in a blender.

Blend until creamy and smooth.

Enjoy chilled.

3. Turmeric Ginger Immune Booster

Ingredients:

1 cup mango chunks

1 small carrot, peeled and chopped

1/2 teaspoon fresh ginger, grated

1/4 teaspoon turmeric powder

1 tablespoon honey

1 cup coconut water

Instructions:
Add all ingredients to a blender.
Blend until smooth and frothy.
Drink immediately.

Tips for Making the Perfect Remission Smoothie

Variety is Key: Rotate ingredients to ensure a wide range of nutrients and avoid monotony.

Stay Hydrated: Incorporate hydrating ingredients like coconut water or cucumbers.

Focus on Freshness: Use fresh, organic ingredients whenever possible to maximize nutrient intake and avoid pesticides.

Listen to Your Body: Adjust recipes based on what feels good and supports your well-being.

Consult Healthcare Providers: Before making significant dietary changes, discuss with your healthcare team to ensure they support your specific health needs.

Smoothies for remission are a delicious and effective way to support ongoing health and prevent cancer recurrence. By incorporating a variety of nutrient-dense ingredients, these smoothies help strengthen the immune system, detoxify the body, and promote overall wellness. They are an easy, enjoyable addition to a healthy lifestyle, helping individuals in remission maintain their strength, vitality, and peace of mind.

Chapter Seven: Smoothies for Various Needs

Detoxifying Smoothies

These delightful drinks are designed to help cleanse the body, flushing out toxins and providing a refreshing boost of nutrients. Detoxifying smoothies can be a fantastic addition to your diet, promoting overall health and vitality in a delicious and convenient way.

Why Detoxifying Smoothies?

In our modern world, we are exposed to various toxins from processed foods, pollution, and even stress. While our bodies are naturally equipped to handle and eliminate these toxins, sometimes they need a little extra help. This is where detoxifying smoothies come in:

Boosting Nutrient Intake: Packed with fruits, vegetables, and superfoods, these smoothies provide essential vitamins and minerals.

Supporting Digestive Health: Ingredients like fiber-rich fruits and vegetables can aid digestion and promote regularity.

Enhancing Energy Levels: By eliminating toxins and supplying clean energy sources, detox smoothies can help you feel more vibrant and energetic.

Promoting Skin Health: Nutrient-rich smoothies can improve skin appearance, giving you a healthy glow.

Supporting Weight Management: These smoothies are often low in calories but high in nutrients, making them great for maintaining a healthy weight.

Key Ingredients for Detoxifying Smoothies

Certain ingredients are particularly effective for detoxification due to their high nutrient content and specific properties.These are some essential components to think about.

Leafy Greens (Spinach, Kale, Swiss Chard): These are packed with chlorophyll, which helps remove toxins from the blood and supports liver function.

Citrus Fruits (Lemons, Oranges, Grapefruits): Rich in vitamin C, these fruits boost the immune system and help flush out toxins.

Ginger: Known for its anti-inflammatory and digestive benefits, ginger aids in detoxifying the body.

Curcumin, a potent antioxidant and anti-inflammatory substance, is found in turmeric.

Beets: These are high in antioxidants and support liver detoxification.

Cucumbers: With high water content, cucumbers help keep you hydrated and flush out toxins.

Apples: High in fiber, apples aid in digestion and help remove toxins from the digestive tract.

Parsley and Cilantro: These herbs help cleanse the kidneys and support the body's natural detox processes.

Chia Seeds: High in fiber and omega-3 fatty acids, chia seeds aid in digestion and provide sustained energy.

Sample Detoxifying Smoothie Recipes

1. Green Detox Smoothie

Ingredients:

1 cup spinach

1/2 cucumber, chopped

1 green apple, cored and chopped

1/2 lemon, juiced

one-inch-long, freshly peeled and grated piece of ginger

1 cup coconut water

Instructions:

Combine all ingredients in a blender.

Blend until smooth.

Serve immediately.

2. Citrus Beet Cleanser

Ingredients:

1 small beet, peeled and chopped

1 orange, peeled and segmented

1/2 lemon, juiced

1 carrot, peeled and chopped

1 cup water or coconut water

Instructions:

Place all ingredients in a blender.

Blend until smooth.

Enjoy chilled.

3. Turmeric Ginger Flush

Ingredients:

1 cup pineapple chunks

1 banana

1/2 teaspoon turmeric powder

one-inch-long, freshly peeled and grated piece of ginger

1 cup almond milk

Instructions:

Add all ingredients to a blender.

Blend until creamy and smooth.

Drink immediately.

Tips for Making the Perfect Detox Smoothie

Use Fresh, Organic Ingredients: To maximize nutrient intake and minimize exposure to pesticides, use fresh, organic fruits and vegetables.

Balance the Flavors: Combine sweet, tart, and earthy flavors to create a delicious and well-rounded smoothie.

Adjust Consistency: Add more liquid (water, coconut water, or almond milk) to achieve your desired smoothie thickness.

Start Slow: If you're new to detox smoothies, start with small portions to see how your body responds.

Stay Hydrated: Drink plenty of water throughout the day to aid in the detoxification process.

Detoxifying smoothies are a fantastic way to support your body's natural cleansing processes while enjoying a delicious and nutritious treat. By including a variety of detoxifying ingredients, you can help flush out toxins, boost your energy, and promote overall health. These smoothies are not only easy to make but also offer a convenient and enjoyable way to enhance your wellness journey. So, grab your blender, mix up some vibrant ingredients, and toast to a healthier, cleaner you.

Smoothies for a Stronger Defense System

Let's explore the concept of smoothies designed to bolster the immune system, particularly in the context of cancer. These smoothies are formulated to strengthen the body's natural defense mechanisms, helping to protect against infections and support overall health during and after cancer treatment.

Why Immune-Boosting Smoothies Matter

Cancer and its treatments, such as chemotherapy and radiation, can significantly weaken the immune system. A compromised immune system leaves the body vulnerable to infections and slows the recovery process. Incorporating immune-boosting smoothies into the diet can provide essential nutrients that enhance the body's ability to fend off illness and promote faster healing.

Key Ingredients for Immune-Boosting Smoothies

The effectiveness of immune-boosting smoothies lies in the selection of ingredients known for their immune-supportive properties. The following are some of the top components to use:

Citrus Fruits (Oranges, Grapefruits, Lemons): High in vitamin C, which is crucial for immune function.

Berries (Strawberries, Blueberries, Raspberries): Packed with antioxidants that protect cells from damage.

Leafy Greens (Spinach, Kale): Rich in vitamins A, C, and K, as well as folate and iron, which support immune health.

Ginger: Known for its anti-inflammatory and antimicrobial properties.

Curcumin, a potent antioxidant and anti-inflammatory substance, is found in turmeric.

Yogurt or Kefir: Provides probiotics that support gut health, which is closely linked to immune function.

Nuts and Seeds (Almonds, Chia Seeds, Flaxseeds): Provide vitamin E and healthy fats that enhance immune responses.

Green tea contains catechins, which have both antiviral and antibacterial activities.

Garlic: Contains allicin, which has immune-boosting properties.

Honey: Known for its antibacterial and soothing properties.

Sample Immune-Boosting Smoothie Recipes

1. Citrus Immune Power Smoothie

Ingredients:

1 orange, peeled and segmented

1/2 grapefruit, peeled and segmented

1/2 lemon, juiced

1 cup spinach

1 tablespoon chia seeds

1 cup green tea (cooled)

Instructions:

Combine all ingredients in a blender.

Blend until smooth.

Serve immediately.

2. Berry Antioxidant Blast

Ingredients:

1/2 cup blueberries

1/2 cup strawberries

1/2 cup raspberries

1/2 cup plain Greek yogurt

1 tablespoon flaxseeds

1 cup almond milk

Instructions:

Place all ingredients in a blender.

Blend until creamy and smooth.

Enjoy chilled.

3. Golden Immunity Smoothie

Ingredients:

1 cup mango chunks

1 banana

1/2 teaspoon turmeric powder

a one-inch-long, freshly peeled and grated piece of ginger

1 tablespoon honey

1 cup coconut water

Instructions:

Add all ingredients to a blender.

Blend until smooth and frothy.

Drink immediately.

Tips for Making Effective Immune-Boosting Smoothies

Choose Fresh, Organic Ingredients: This maximizes nutrient content and minimizes exposure to pesticides and other harmful substances.

Balance the Flavors: Combining sweet, tart, and earthy flavors can make your smoothie both nutritious and delicious.

Adjust Consistency: Use more or less liquid to achieve your preferred smoothie thickness.

Listen to Your Body: Tailor ingredients to what your body needs and tolerates well.

Stay Hydrated: Adequate hydration is key to supporting immune function, so make sure your smoothies contribute to your daily fluid intake.

Immune-boosting smoothies can be a valuable part of a cancer patient's diet, offering a delicious and easy way to support the body's natural defense system. By incorporating ingredients rich in vitamins, antioxidants, and other immune-supportive compounds, these smoothies can help strengthen resilience against infections and promote overall health. Whether you are undergoing treatment, in recovery, or in remission, these nutrient-packed smoothies can play a crucial role in maintaining your strength and vitality. So, grab your blender, experiment with different ingredients, and enjoy the nourishing benefits of these powerful drinks.

Maintaining a Healthy Lifestyle: Smoothies as a Daily Routine

In the journey of maintaining a healthy lifestyle, especially when faced with the challenges of cancer, incorporating smoothies into your daily routine can be a game-changer. These nutrient-rich blends offer a simple, convenient, and enjoyable way to ensure your body gets the essential vitamins, minerals, and antioxidants it needs to fight off illness, support recovery, and promote overall well-being.

Smoothies are incredibly versatile, allowing you to tailor each blend to meet your specific nutritional needs and preferences. For cancer patients and survivors, this means you can create smoothies that are packed with ingredients known for their cancer-fighting properties, as well as those that help manage treatment side effects and boost your immune system.

The Power of Consistency
One of the key benefits of making smoothies a daily habit is the consistency it brings to your nutritional intake. When you commit to drinking a smoothie every day, you're more likely to consume a balanced array of nutrients regularly. This is crucial for cancer patients,

whose bodies often need extra support to cope with the stress of treatments like chemotherapy and radiation.

By starting your day with a smoothie, you set a positive tone for the rest of your meals. It's a proactive step towards nourishing your body, helping to stabilize blood sugar levels, and providing sustained energy throughout the day. Moreover, the act of preparing and enjoying a smoothie can become a comforting ritual, offering a sense of normalcy and control during a time that can often feel chaotic.

Building Nutrient-Dense Smoothies

The foundation of a health-boosting smoothie lies in its ingredients. Focus on incorporating a variety of fruits and vegetables, particularly those rich in antioxidants, vitamins, and minerals. Berries, such as blueberries, strawberries, and raspberries, are excellent choices due to their high antioxidant content, which helps protect cells from damage. Leafy greens, like spinach and kale, are high in vitamins A, C, and K, as well as folate and fiber.

Adding a source of healthy fats, such as avocado, nuts, or seeds, can enhance the absorption of fat-soluble vitamins and provide a sense of satiety. Proteins are also crucial, especially for those undergoing cancer treatment, as they aid in tissue repair and immune function. Greek yogurt, protein powders, or nut butters can be great additions to your smoothie to ensure you get an adequate protein intake.

Detoxifying and Immune-Boosting Ingredients

Detoxifying ingredients can help your body eliminate toxins, potentially reducing the burden on your liver and kidneys. Ingredients like lemon, ginger, turmeric, and beets are known for their detoxifying properties. Turmeric, in particular, contains curcumin, which has been studied for its anti-inflammatory and anticancer effects.

Immune-boosting ingredients are also vital for cancer patients. Citrus fruits, such as oranges and lemons, are high in vitamin C, which supports immune function. Probiotic-rich ingredients like kefir or yogurt can help maintain a healthy gut microbiome, which is closely linked to immune health. Additionally, ingredients like garlic and green tea have compounds that can enhance the immune response.

Adapting to Treatment Side Effects
Cancer treatments can often bring a host of side effects, including nausea, loss of appetite,

and digestive issues. Smoothies can be adapted to help manage these symptoms. For example, ginger and peppermint are well-known for their ability to reduce nausea. Blending these into a smoothie with soothing ingredients like banana and almond milk can create a gentle, stomach-friendly drink.

If you struggle with appetite loss, nutrient-dense smoothies can provide essential calories and nutrients without requiring you to eat large meals. They can be sipped slowly throughout the day, ensuring you receive the necessary nourishment even when solid foods are unappealing.

A Sustainable Health Practice
Incorporating smoothies into your daily routine is not just a short-term strategy but a sustainable health practice. It encourages a lifelong habit of prioritizing nutrition and

self-care. This is particularly important for cancer survivors, who must remain vigilant about their health to reduce the risk of recurrence and support long-term recovery.

Making smoothies a daily ritual also offers a creative outlet. Experimenting with different ingredients, flavors, and textures can be enjoyable and empowering. It allows you to take an active role in your health, making informed choices about what you consume.

Maintaining a healthy lifestyle, particularly in the context of cancer, involves a holistic approach to nutrition and self-care. Smoothies provide an accessible, versatile, and enjoyable way to incorporate essential nutrients into your diet. By making them a daily routine, you can support your body's healing processes, boost your immune system, and improve your overall quality of life.

Remember, the route to better health is composed of tiny, persistent steps. Starting your day with a nutrient-packed smoothie can be one of the most impactful habits you adopt, offering a daily dose of wellness in a delicious, convenient package. Accept the power of smoothies and take a proactive approach to a better, stronger self.

Chapter Eight

Smoothies for Specific Cancer Types

Let's explore the idea of smoothies designed for particular cancer kinds.. These smoothies are designed to address the unique nutritional needs and symptoms associated with different cancers. By customizing ingredients, we can better support the body's requirements and enhance the healing process. Here, we'll explore smoothies tailored for breast cancer, prostate cancer, colorectal cancer, and lung cancer.

Smoothies for Breast Cancer

Breast cancer patients often benefit from foods rich in antioxidants, phytoestrogens, and anti-inflammatory compounds. These ingredients can help manage side effects from treatment and support overall health.

Key Ingredients:

Berries (Blueberries, Strawberries): High in antioxidants that combat oxidative stress.

Flaxseeds: Contain lignans, which have been shown to have anti-cancer properties.

Leafy Greens (Spinach, Kale): Packed with vitamins and minerals that support the immune system.

Green Tea: Rich in catechins, which may help inhibit cancer cell growth.

Turmeric: Known for its powerful anti-inflammatory effects.

Sample Recipe:Berry Antioxidant Smoothie

Ingredients:

1/2 cup blueberries

1/2 cup strawberries

1 tablespoon ground flaxseeds

1 cup spinach

1 cup green tea (cooled)

1/2 teaspoon turmeric

Instructions:

Combine all ingredients in a blender.

Blend until smooth.

Serve immediately.

Smoothies for Prostate Cancer

For prostate cancer, foods rich in lycopene, antioxidants, and omega-3 fatty acids are particularly beneficial. These nutrients can help manage inflammation and support prostate health.

Key Ingredients:

Tomatoes: High in lycopene, which may help reduce prostate cancer risk.

Pomegranate: Contains antioxidants that support overall health.

Walnuts: Provide omega-3 fatty acids, which have anti-inflammatory properties.

Broccoli: Contains the anti-cancer substance sulforaphane.

Berries: Rich in antioxidants.

Sample Recipe: Lycopene Power Smoothie

Ingredients:

1 medium tomato, chopped

1/2 cup pomegranate seeds

1/2 cup blueberries

1/4 cup walnuts

1/2 cup broccoli florets

1 cup water

Instructions:

Add all ingredients to a blender.

Blend until smooth.

Enjoy chilled.

Smoothies for Colorectal Cancer

For colorectal cancer, it's important to focus on ingredients that promote gut health, provide fiber, and have anti-inflammatory properties.

These can help with digestion and support overall well-being.

Key Ingredients:

Oats: High in fiber, which supports digestive health.

Bananas: Gentle on the stomach and provide potassium.

Ginger: Helps with nausea and has anti-inflammatory effects.

Kefir: Provides probiotics for gut health.

Carrots: High in beta-carotene, which has antioxidant properties.

Sample Recipe: Digestive Health Smoothie

Ingredients:

1/2 cup rolled oats

1 banana

1/2 teaspoon fresh ginger, grated

1 cup kefir

1 medium carrot, peeled and chopped

1 cup water

Instructions:

Place all ingredients in a blender.

Blend until smooth.

Serve immediately.

Smoothies for Lung Cancer

Lung cancer patients can benefit from smoothies rich in vitamins A and C, antioxidants, and anti-inflammatory compounds. These nutrients help support lung health and overall immunity.

Key Ingredients:

Carrots: High in beta-carotene, which is beneficial for lung health.

Oranges: Rich in vitamin C, which supports the immune system.

Ginger: Reduces inflammation and aids in digestion.

Turmeric: Has powerful anti-inflammatory effects.

Leafy Greens (Kale, Spinach): Packed with vitamins and minerals.

Sample Recipe: Lung Health Smoothie

Ingredients:

1 medium carrot, peeled and chopped

1 orange, peeled and segmented

1/2 teaspoon fresh ginger, grated

1/4 teaspoon turmeric

1 cup kale

1 cup water or coconut water

Instructions:

Combine all ingredients in a blender.

Blend until smooth.

Drink immediately.

General Tips for Making Cancer-Specific Smoothies

Customize to Preferences: Adjust recipes based on what tastes good and what your body tolerates well.

Use Fresh, Organic Ingredients: This ensures maximum nutrient intake and reduces exposure to harmful chemicals.

Balance Nutrients: Include a mix of fruits, vegetables, proteins, and healthy fats to create a balanced smoothie.

Listen to Your Body: Pay attention to how different ingredients make you feel and adjust accordingly.

Emotional and Psychological Benefits

Creating and consuming these smoothies can also provide emotional and psychological benefits. The act of preparing a nutrient-rich smoothie can offer a sense of control and empowerment during a challenging time. Enjoying a delicious, colorful smoothie can lift spirits and provide a moment of pleasure, contributing positively to overall well-being.

Smoothies tailored for specific cancer types offer a personalized approach to nutrition that can support healing and long-term health. By selecting ingredients that address the unique needs and challenges associated with each type of cancer, these smoothies can play a crucial role in maintaining strength, boosting immunity, and promoting overall wellness.

Conclusion

"Smoothies for Cancer" is a journey into the powerful intersection of nutrition and health, particularly in the context of battling cancer. This book is designed to be a beacon of hope and a practical guide for those navigating the challenges of cancer, whether you are a patient, a survivor, or someone aiming to reduce their risk.

Cancer is a complex disease that requires a comprehensive approach to treatment and recovery. While medical interventions are critical, the role of diet in supporting the body's natural defenses and promoting healing cannot be overstated. Smoothies, with their versatility and nutrient density, emerge as an exceptional tool in this regard. They offer an easy and enjoyable way to deliver a concentrated dose of vitamins, minerals, antioxidants, and other bioactive compounds known for their cancer-fighting properties.

The recipes and guidance provided are crafted with care, keeping in mind the unique needs of those affected by cancer. Whether you are looking to boost your immune system, manage treatment side effects, or support your recovery, there is a smoothie recipe to help you on your journey. The beauty of smoothies lies in their adaptability—they can be tailored to fit individual tastes and dietary requirements, ensuring that everyone can find joy and benefit in this nutritious habit.

Making smoothies a daily routine offers consistency, which is key to reaping long-term health benefits. By starting your day with a nutrient-packed smoothie, you set a positive tone for the rest of your meals, helping to stabilize blood sugar levels, provide sustained energy, and foster a sense of empowerment over your health. This simple daily practice can become a comforting ritual, offering not only physical nourishment but also emotional support during trying times.

This book underscores the importance of integrating good nutrition into your daily life as a sustainable and enjoyable way to support your overall well-being. This commitment to healthy eating is particularly important for cancer survivors, who must remain vigilant about their health to support long-term recovery and reduce the risk of recurrence.

Ultimately, this book aims to empower you with knowledge and practical tools to take an active role in your health journey. Preparing and enjoying smoothies can be a powerful act of self-care, allowing you to make informed choices about what you consume and how you nourish your body. Each smoothie you create and consume is a step towards a healthier, stronger you.

In conclusion, "Smoothies for Cancer" is a testament to the healing potential of nutrition. We hope this book inspires you to explore the vibrant world of smoothies and to make them a part of your daily routine. By doing so, you can harness the power of food to support your body in the fight against cancer, boost your immune system, and enhance your overall quality of life.